THIS MUCH I KNOW

Written by Heather Barnard

Art by Eva Magill-Oliver

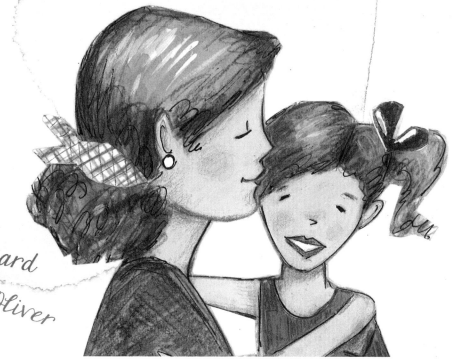

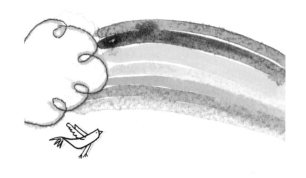

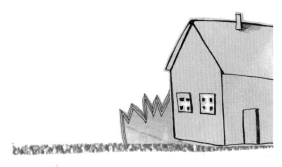

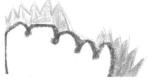

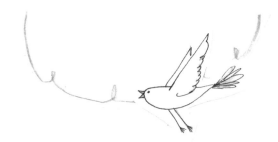

For you mom, because I know in my heart that you knew all along, just how much I love you. And for giving me a world filled with pink linings on every cloud. I'll always remember tacos for Christmas Day dinner, rubber duckies on rainy days, Donald Duck talk, cuddles in overstuffed chairs and forever being a child at heart.

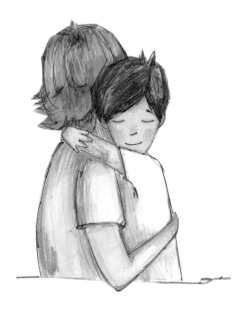

"This much I know, this much is true,
I'll always remember, I was loved by you."

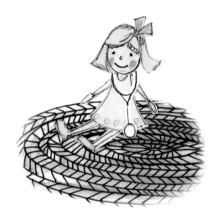

Children all over the world are feeling just like you. Their mommies have cancer too, and the little girls and boys each have so many questions and fears inside. They have questions they want to ask, but aren't sure how. Some children are afraid to talk about cancer...are you? Some children want to know what is going to happen to their mommy...do you? The children in this story are here to help you know that all the questions and feelings you have are all okay. They have them too. They want to show you that no matter what, you will always feel your mommy by your side.

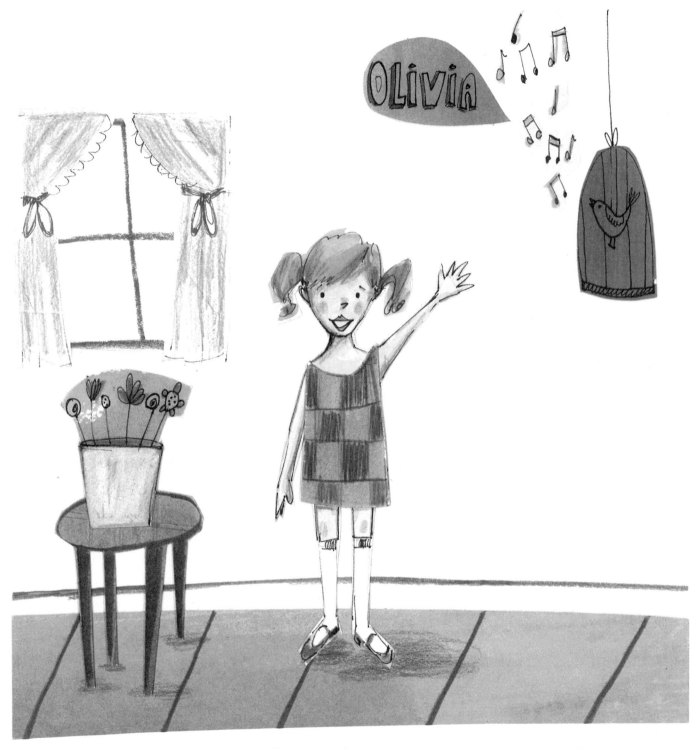

Meet Olivia! Olivia is a funny little girl who loves to giggle and play.

But Olivia's smile has been a little topsy-turvy lately...
she found out her mommy has cancer, and now she doesn't know what to feel.
Do you know how Olivia feels? I bet she feels just like you.

"I'm feeling quite sad, I'm feeling quite blue.
My mommy is sick, what should I do?"

After worrying and thinking, Olivia finally
asked her mommy this,

"Mommy, will you be ok?"

Her mommy scooped Olivia up in her arms,
swung her around and whispered these words:

"This much I know, whatever's ahead,
you'll still feel my kisses on your sweet
little forehead."

Olivia let out the little
giggle and grin her mommy
was used to.

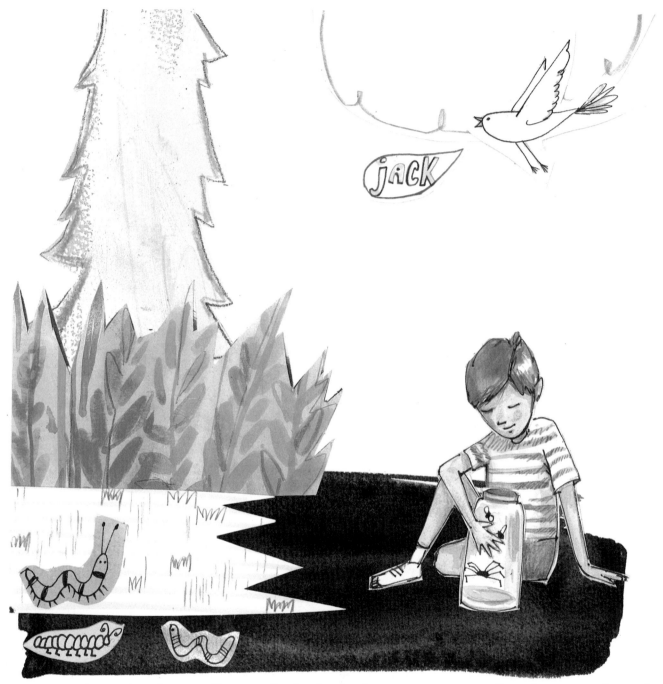

This is Jack! He's a bug collector. Jack always has a worm or a beetle or a roly-poly in his pocket. Do you like collecting icky bugs? Jack likes to sit in the yard with his bugs and think about his mommy. She is sick too.

What's wrong with my mommy? I can tell she's not well. How do I talk to my mommy?
I have so much to tell. Jack would do anything to make his mommy smile and he thought
of just the way to do it.

"Mommy, do you know I love you from here up to the littlest planet and back?"

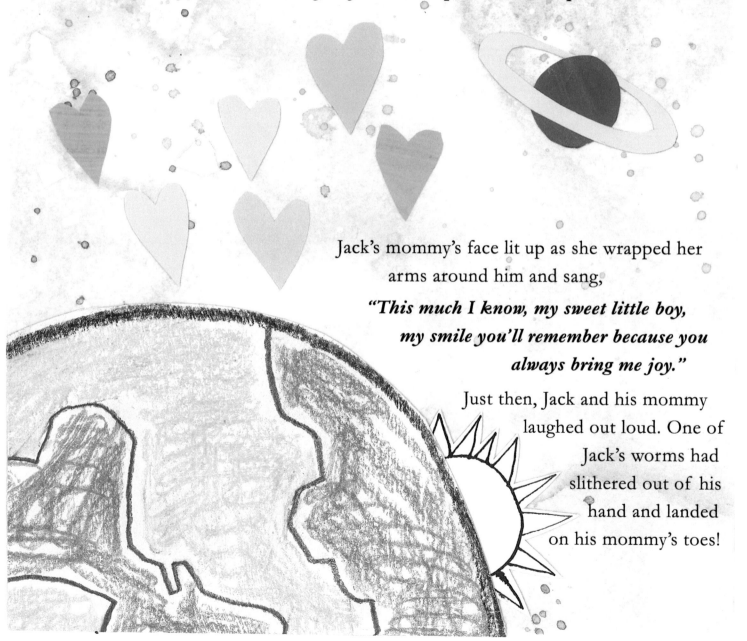

Jack's mommy's face lit up as she wrapped her
arms around him and sang,

*"This much I know, my sweet little boy,
my smile you'll remember because you
always bring me joy."*

Just then, Jack and his mommy
laughed out loud. One of
Jack's worms had
slithered out of his
hand and landed
on his mommy's toes!

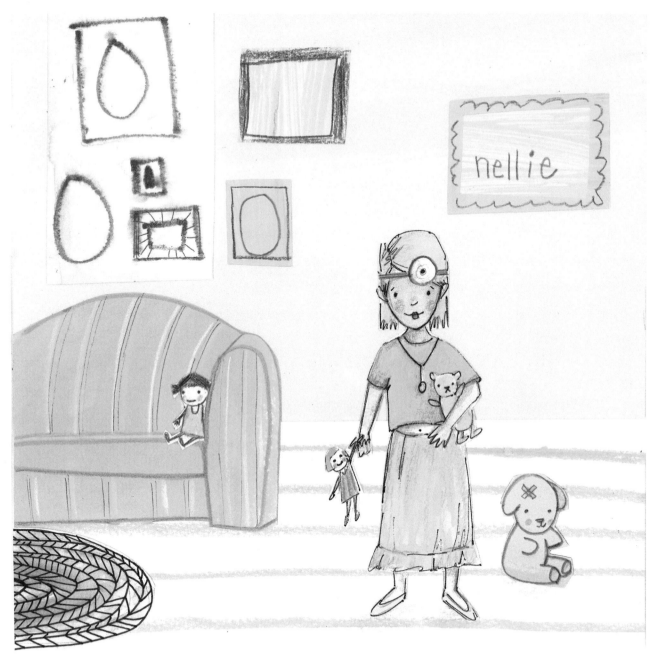

Sweet little Nellie is a caring person at heart. She likes to play doctor with her dollies and stuffed animals. She gives them shots, takes their temperatures, and gives them lots of kisses and hugs. She cares about her mommy very much too, and wonders what happens at her mommy's doctor visits. Do you wonder this too?

My mommy has cancer, and goes to the doctor a lot.

I wonder what cancer feels like, does she have to get a shot?

Above all, Nellie wants her mommy to know that she cares for her too. So she asked her mommy,

"Mommy, do you need me to hold your hand when you're scared at the doctor's office?"

Nellie's mommy was overjoyed at the sweetness of her little girl. She held her tight and said,

"This much I know, our love will flow. Sometimes I'll be scared, but I'll know how much you cared."

Nellie took out her little doctor kit and started taking care of her mommy, just like her dollies, with the same special care.

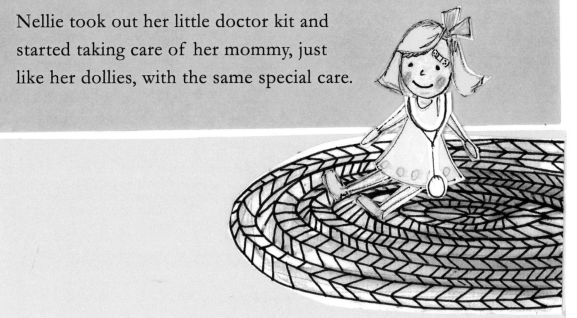

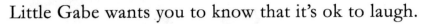

Little Gabe wants you to know that it's ok to laugh.

Gabe turned something he thought was scary into something funny.

Do you do funny things with your mom?

Mom's hair is falling out. She wears all kinds of wigs. I think they're kind of fun.

Hey mom, do you like my new digs?

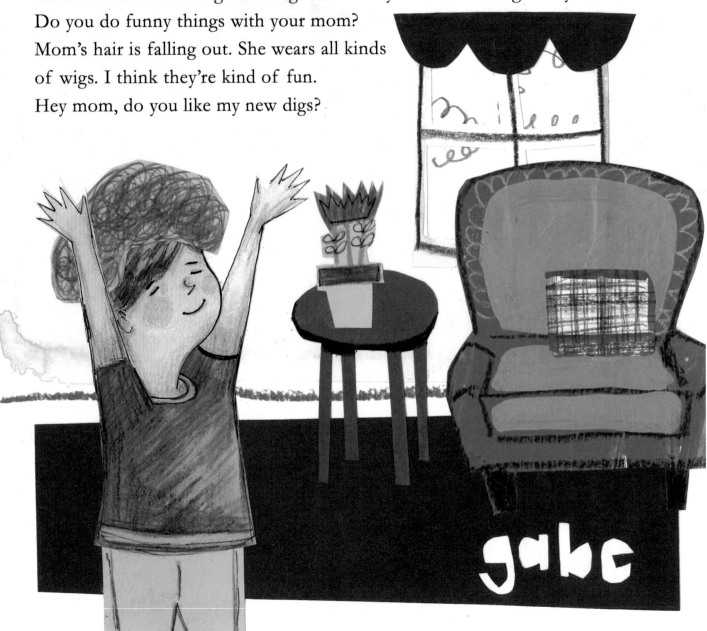

gabe

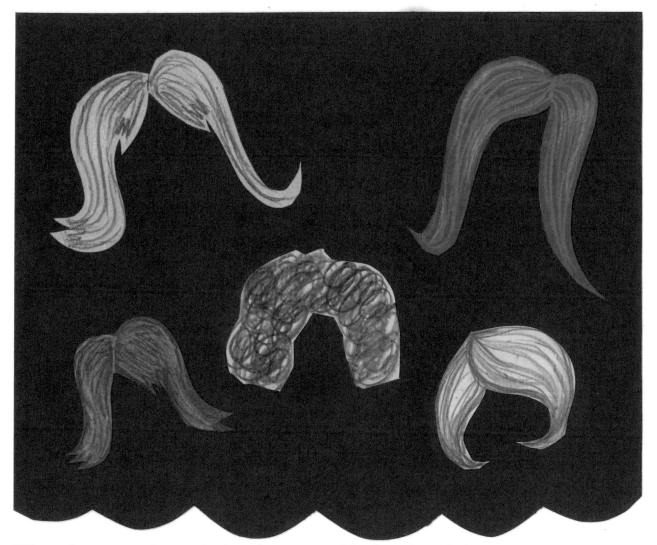

When they were done playing dress-up with the wigs, Gabe's mom took hers off. When Gabe saw her bald head he asked,

"Mom, will we always have this much fun together?"

His mom smiled down with soft spoken eyes and reminded him of this:

**"This much I know, my funny little man,
we can always play pretend, even if with you, I cannot stand."**

Gabe hugged his mom tight and then placed the wig with long, flowing locks on her head. Then his mom put a curly wig on him and together they laughed and played.

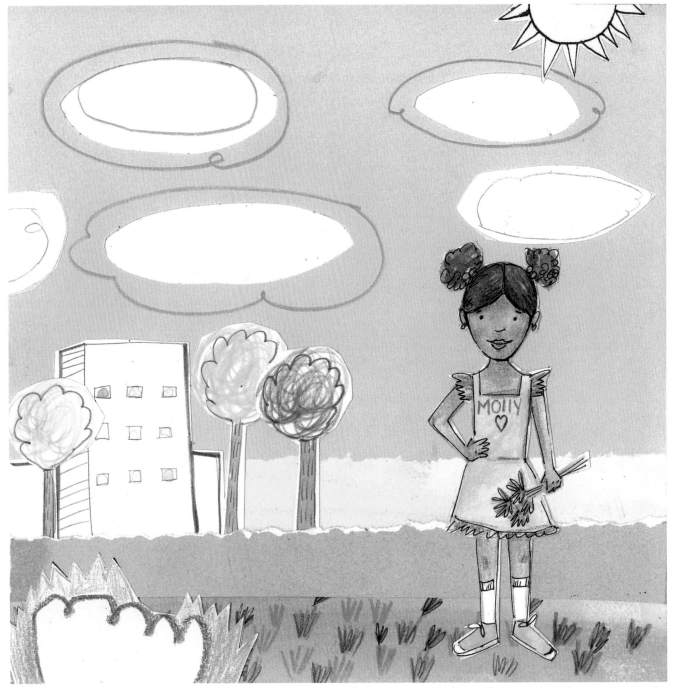

Eight-year-old Molly doesn't know what a hospital is like, do you? She knows her mommy has to go there, sometimes for long stays. She's a little afraid of what might happen there. Does your mommy have to go to a hospital too?

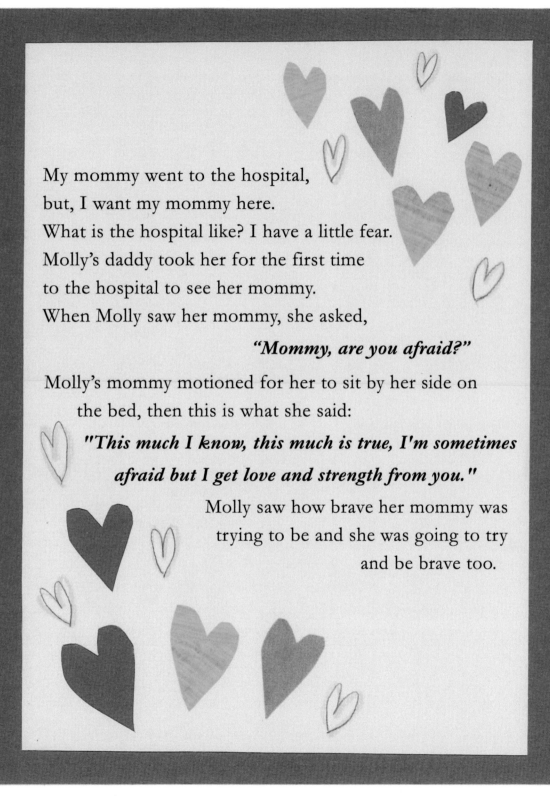

My mommy went to the hospital,
but, I want my mommy here.
What is the hospital like? I have a little fear.
Molly's daddy took her for the first time
to the hospital to see her mommy.
When Molly saw her mommy, she asked,

"Mommy, are you afraid?"

Molly's mommy motioned for her to sit by her side on
the bed, then this is what she said:

**"This much I know, this much is true, I'm sometimes
afraid but I get love and strength from you."**

Molly saw how brave her mommy was
trying to be and she was going to try
and be brave too.

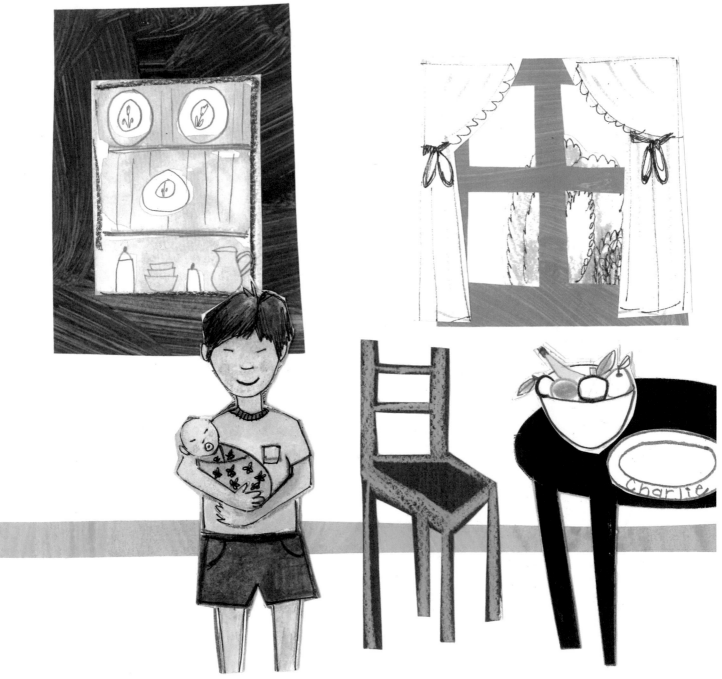

Charlie is the oldest of his brothers and sisters. He's always taking care of them and helping out. Since his mom is sick, he helps even more. He can see his mom is weak.

Do you help your mom with
your brothers and sisters?
He remembers the special moments
he has with his mom alone.

My mom is my best friend.
She's the greatest person there is.
I like to do everything with mom, even giggle
over soda pop fizz.

Charlie looked at his mom, lying on the couch,
and he needed to know,

"Mommy, will you still share your special time with me?"

His mom raised her head and sat up tall, then held him
close and told him this:

*"This much I know, you'll always remember,
those times I sang to you as you fell
to your slumber."*

Charlie sat in his mom's arms while she rocked
him back and forth, singing her special song.
Charlie smiled; he loves these times with mom.

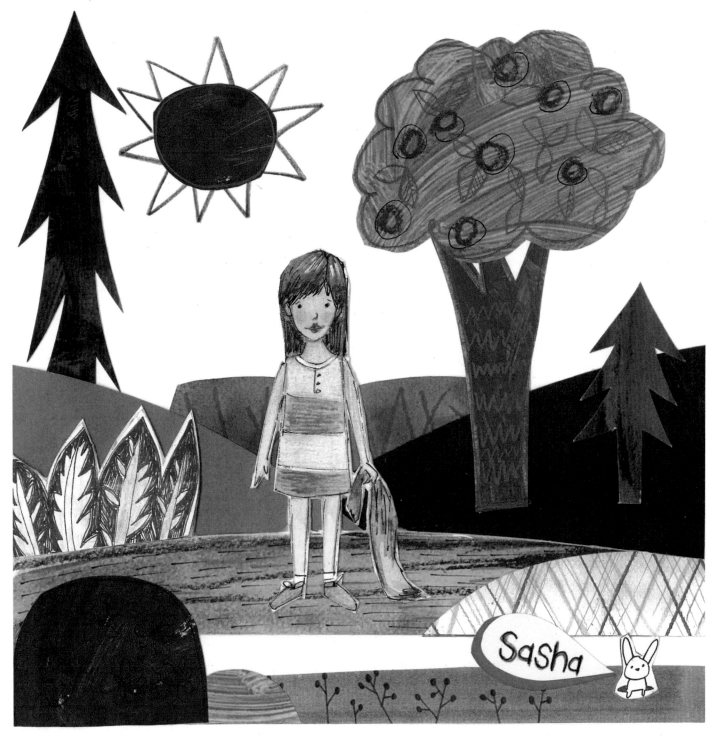

Sasha has a favorite purple blanket that she takes everywhere she goes.

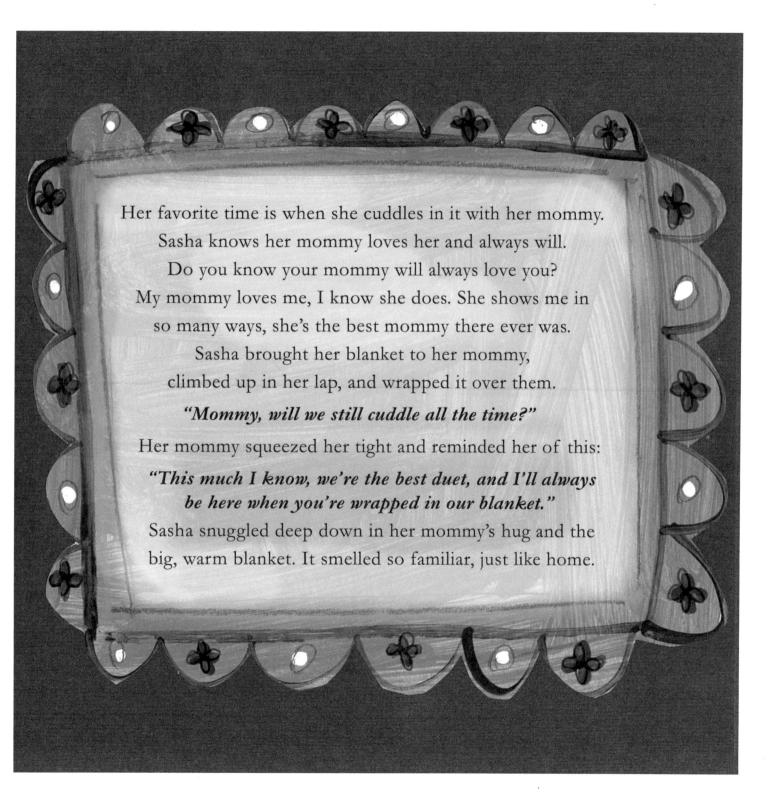

Her favorite time is when she cuddles in it with her mommy.
Sasha knows her mommy loves her and always will.
Do you know your mommy will always love you?
My mommy loves me, I know she does. She shows me in
so many ways, she's the best mommy there ever was.
Sasha brought her blanket to her mommy,
climbed up in her lap, and wrapped it over them.

"Mommy, will we still cuddle all the time?"

Her mommy squeezed her tight and reminded her of this:

**"This much I know, we're the best duet, and I'll always
be here when you're wrapped in our blanket."**

Sasha snuggled deep down in her mommy's hug and the
big, warm blanket. It smelled so familiar, just like home.

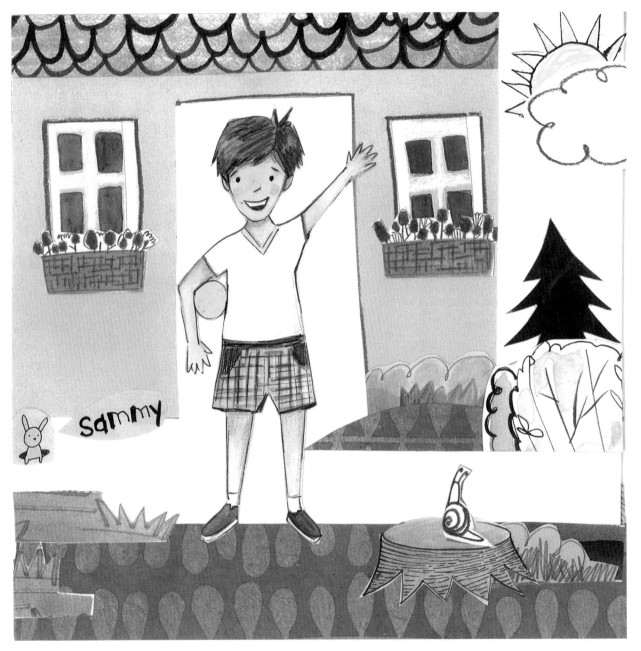

Sammy hopes that you've heard his friends and been comforted by what they have said. They know you have lots of questions, because they do too.

Sammy wants you to always remember this: *"I talk to my mommy and tell her how I feel. It's ok to be scared when you love someone a great deal."*

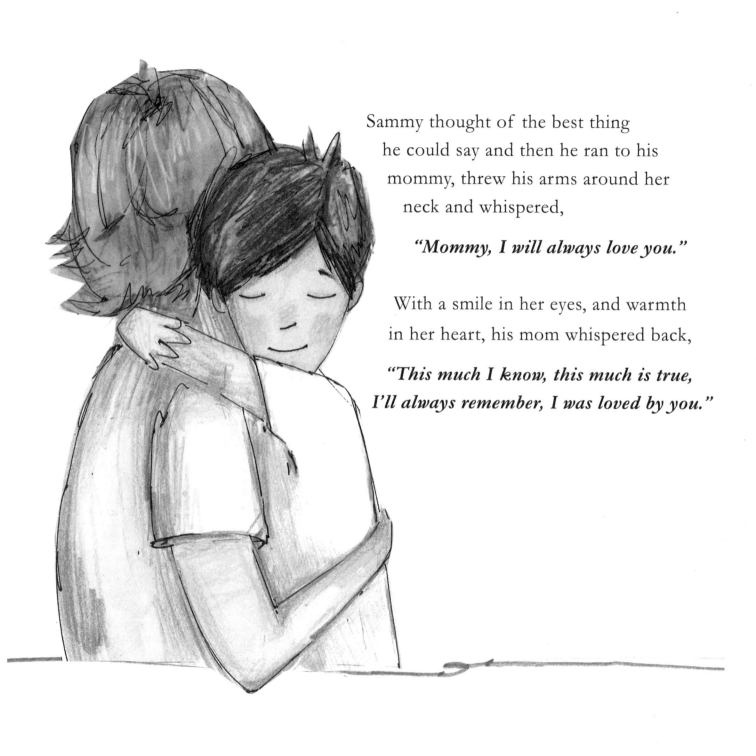

Sammy thought of the best thing he could say and then he ran to his mommy, threw his arms around her neck and whispered,

"Mommy, I will always love you."

With a smile in her eyes, and warmth in her heart, his mom whispered back,

"This much I know, this much is true, I'll always remember, I was loved by you."

Kids: Write or draw your questions for mom
or details of your favorite times spent together.

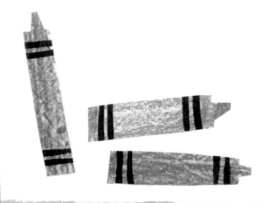

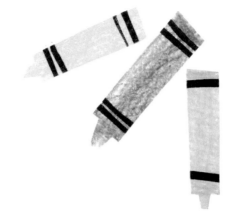

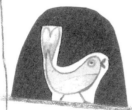

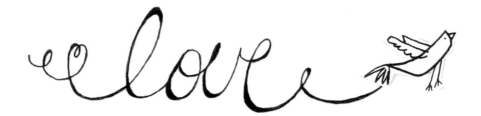

Parents: This much I know...

_____

_____

_____

_____

_____

_____

_____

_____

_____

_____

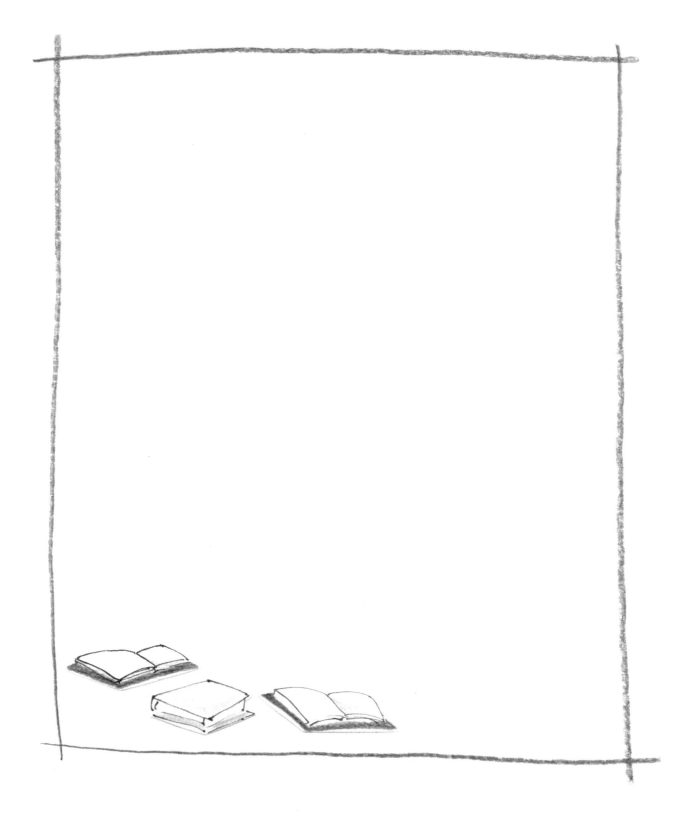

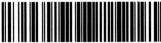